"Tribute to the dead, but don't ask to join."

ACKNOWLEDGMENT:

This work did not receive any funding. The original concept of this review was to answer the question of how to have an entirely home-based solution for COVID19. But in due course, as the study progressed, the concept of problem-solving like value innovation, functional fixation of things, were utilized. And this web search was evolved into this form. With a basic understanding of health itself being altered to find solutions to COVID 19 problem of death, during the pre-vaccination time, and the principle of treatments like benefits outweighs harm; rather unconventional reasoning is established. "If it's possible to solve a puzzle if only a few pieces know, the pieces still unidentified will fill vacant places on their own. The parameters must be limited in a closed space, as the human body is a closed space, there is left a lot of blank space, to be filled on its own with regular diet." This review paper is intended to serve as a framework for universal therapy. This book also explores new methods of clinical testing as it is not ideal to be dependent on genetics alone when health status is evaluated. The theory is probably still incomplete, and someone with proper resources will confirm and advance this theory. Rahul Tiwari and Vinayak Raj, I will like to thank you for your occasional consult on how to write a paper but still couldn't publish it in the journal. Lastly, an apology as deductions is considered unethical in medical science.

-Dr. Vivek Kumar

Chapter 1: The COVID problem

COVID is spreading fast, and getting infected is a problem, but not the entire/precise problem. The entire problem comprises a spectrum of the problem. Namely, beginning with mortality or simply a possibility of death is the most important and dreadful. A bit less serious is the disability, which may be temporary or permanent with or without any event of death. The third type, where symptoms are present and the patient gets by just fine with simple medications/treatment. The fourth type is least dangerous with the infection without symptoms. A doctor doesn't want you to die as it is the worst-case scenario, regardless of whether you contract COVID infection or not. Regarding infection, since it spreads fast don't get infected. And if still, you get infected; in descending order of priorities based on outcomes, avoid mortality, avoid disability, have the least discomfort during the infectivity period. All four of them can lead to complications, but all infections have to be one of the four, and we can try decreasing the severity, a level down, then so we can try solving the COVID problem.

COVID infection shows higher toxic insult and bad outcomes in patients with co-morbidities, especially old age. Science classifies aging as a pathological process, and to date, it is not possible to reverse aging. However, aging unlike other risk factors exhibits association in multiples of thousands to different diseases. A minor alteration may provide an efficient solution to the COVID problem.

The COVID pandemic is showing the majority of cases healing on its own, with mild to no distress. A general approach has been to increase immunity to decrease the severity of disease if infected. However, immunity is just a body function, and it can be improved further if the entire body function is improved.

A peak human body would not require an outside environment but rather its system to survive, like an ecosystem. It can be interpreted to be said as," the net changes a body could undergo would be net-zero (ex: healing its damages while recovering 100% functionality), would be an ideal peak human body. But this is the sound of fiction.

A more realistic approach would be attaining
a) best physiological state, with
b) exogenous attenuation of residual negative changes.
The best physiological state without exterior intervention should be healthy aging, and the closest description of such is with the MARK-AGE project. The intention is to attain the most synergistic aging to a human capacity.

Mathematically,
$$(\text{biological age} \approx \text{chronological age});$$
or, $(\text{biological age} < \text{chronological age})$, if possible.

In terms of lay parlance, immunity hasn't been scalable, nor a physiological functioning standard. We do have normal physiological limits that any doctor co-relates with their clinical findings. So to attain the best possible scenario of body function, considering aging to be a biological process, and approach as to how much a person can do to avoid severity in case of COVID19.

Chapter 2: Age and Aging

Your age is the time duration from the moment of birth to the present when you are reading it, called chronological age. You cannot change it. Changing it is called time travel. And we all know people of the same age group with different health statuses, ranging from the verge of death to the peak of health. This is called the biological age. It is not a function of time and can be changed. Aging is the process of change of biological age; or, an accumulation of metabolic waste that impairs bodily function to maintain physiological normal is called aging. So, your biological age is the sum of all previous impairments accumulated and the current aging rate. We also cannot change the previous impairments significantly through external interventions. And the rate of aging isn't constant throughout life, it is changing. The current rate of aging is metabolic waste generation and a major portion is a redox-mediated impairment. Thus anti-oxidant-based interventions are lowering metabolic waste generation and the rate of aging. This consequently will reduce the biological age of a person and approach lower chronological age.

For instance, if a chronologically aged 40 years person functions as a biologically aged 40 years old, the person is healthy enough. Now for the same chronological age (i.e. 40 years) if one has a biological age less than 40 years, healthier than the previous instance.

And regarding pre-existing accumulated metabolic wastes there is an intrinsic ability to heal, and supplementing decreased rate of generation of this metabolic waste, clearance of accumulated metabolic waste and repair of consecutive impairments improves.

Chapter 3: MARK – AGE PROJECT

In the year 2013, in an attempt to establish correlation and formulate biological biomarkers based formula for the age of a person, a large scale European study was concluded. It started in 2008. They studied families whose offsprings had a longer life span in comparison to the normal population; called them genetical offsprings of long-living individuals (GO). They also studied spouses of genetic offsprings (SGO), and young adults and old aged people of the normal population, on the same standards.

Alexander Bürkle, the lead scientist of this project published a paper titled, "Associations between Specific Redox Biomarkers and Age in a Large European Cohort: The MARK-AGE Project." His findings included three antioxidants and two redox biomarkers. Antioxidant lycopene is lower in the older population as well as in offspring of longer living individuals (GO) and their spouses (SGO). GO and SGO also exhibits higher levels of cysteine and α-tocopherol. And among redox biomarkers, lower malondialdehyde and higher 3-nitrotyrosine levels are present. These findings need discussion after interpretation. Here only the interpretation of these findings has been presented.

Lycopene —As it's possible to affect its serum levels, proven by lower lycopene levels in SGO lower lycopene level in favor of longevity is a dietary/behavioral intervention. Now maintaining lower levels of lycopene is simply decreased uptake of lycopene, decrease in consumption. However, the older age group from the normal population also has lower lycopene levels and these individuals are not our standard reference of health. Lycopene is not classified as an essential nutrient but is an excellent antioxidant, taken mostly from diet and with age, its gut absorption decreases. Both the facts mentioned contradict each other, it would only make sense if the increased utility of lycopene is based on behavioral/dietary activity in GO and SGO, saturating the lycopene utility pathway, lowering plasma lycopene levels. So, increased consumption of a lycopene-based diet complemented with dietary/behavioral interventions promotes lycopene metabolism.

Cysteine and α-tocopherol plasma levels are high in offsprings of the long-living individuals (GO) and their spouses (SGO). Similar to the lycopene, we can give dietary intervention, to increase their plasma level.

Malondialdehyde in offspring of long-living individuals shows low plasma levels, and it is unrelated to the plasma level of their spouses (SGO), so it is a genetic adaptation. It will be the limiting factor probably, but the most important one, thus a genetic mimicry, through diet and behavior to lower it as much as possible.

3- Nitro tyrosine increased in descendants of long-living individuals (GO) only, thus a genetic adaptation. It's a product of tyrosine nitration, so an increased serum level would indicate: either more tyrosine nitration, via different or one tyrosine nitration pathway, or decreased 3-nitro tyrosine catabolism.

These antioxidants and biomarkers also show interaction among themselves. Here we have lower lycopene, higher vitamin E levels; and lycopene show interaction by repairing vitamin E radical, and product of this reaction can be repaired by vitamin C, under the following reactions:-

Lycopene + TOH+˙ → TOH + Lycopene+
Lycopene+˙ + ASCH2 → Lycopene + ASCH˙ + H+
Lycopene+˙ + ASCH- → Lycopene + ASCH˙- + H+

	3-Nitrotyrosine	Malondialdehyde
Lycopene	↓↓ (free radical scavenging)	↓↓ (free radical scavenging)
Cysteine	↓↓↓ (peroxynitrite mediated)	↓ (via BCL2)
α-tocopherol	↓ (Indirectly via lycopene)	↓ (Indirectly via lycopene + free radical scavenging)

TABLE 2: INTERACTION BETWEEN REDOX MARKERS OF MARK AGE PROJECT

Further, lower 3-nitrotyrosine, levels can be achieved by higher cysteine, tocopherol, and lycopene (free radical scavenging activity of lycopene) consumption.

However, another goal of the MARK-AGE project to gain insight into anti-aging interventions, as clinical regimen, or as diet, remains unfulfilled as no specific paper indicating/compiling the findings of the MARK-AGE project as a diet or clinical regimen. Here, a correlation between redox markers with age has been discussed.

Chapter 4: Lycopene

LYCOPENE: A major carotenoid in human plasma and tissue of linear carotene group. It shows high tolerance, low toxicity, and antioxidant function. Still classified as a non-essential nutrient, it doesn't have any recommended daily dose.[1,2] However, it shows an increase in plasma levels after a five-day meal,[1] and increased antioxidant activity with olive oil consumption.[2] Also, lycopene supplementation in carotenoid deficient older individuals shows an enormous health impact, which favors earlier interpretation. Oral lycopene supplementation alone shows an increase in plasma lycopene levels but no improvement in plasma antioxidant activity is seen.[3] Lycopene supplementation on two biomarkers of lipid peroxidation namely LDL oxidizability, and urinary F2-isoprostanes shows no effect.[4] A study showing medium-dose oral lycopene supplementation is more beneficial than high dose indicates limiting factors. The beneficial effect of tomato with olive oil, especially increased bioavailability,[3] may be augmentations of limiting factors helping in lycopene bioavailability. These findings are in favor of an earlier interpretation of the existence of a dietary complementary factor, which may or may not present in the food sources of lycopene. So proceeding with the deduction of multifactorial metabolic catabolism, higher uptake of lycopene will be the first step; and consumption of dietary complementing factors, second.

DIETARY INDICATION-

1) Sources- Tomato,[3] raw papaya fruit,[5] carrots, watermelon.[6]
2) Bioavailability: Poor bioavailability as a single diet, is not sufficient to raise lycopene levels, but five-day consumption showed increased lycopene levels.[2,4] It has poorer bioavailability in old age,[1] so taking up with probiotics may be helpful. Bioavailability is also subject to heating, lycopene is heat sensitive, and at the same time show trans to cis isomerization and cis-isomer is highly bioavailable. Heating is recommended with olive oil.[7] Heating tomato with onion and olive oil for 2 hours showed z-isomerization which is highly bioavailable.[7]
3) Cuisines:
    a) Tomato-onion-olive oil puree heated for 2 hours[7]
    b) Watermelon consumption, twice per week,[6]
    c) chop tomatoes into 16 small pieces, and heat with olive oil, for at least 10 mins, cis-isomerization increases with heating, at 1 hour it shows the highest cis-form (>90%), so a choice is dependent on users[3]
    d) Air-dried tomatoes>sun dried tomatoes[2]
    e) raw papaya fruit consumption, one serving each day in 1st week, then alternate days from 2nd week.[5]
4) Dietary approaches helping lycopene function: Vitamin C-rich fruit (discussed below), thrice per day 8 hours apart.[8]

5) The dose recommended: High dose lycopene for 5 days, once or twice a month, along with vitamin C-rich food thrice daily, during high dose lycopene period followed by low dose lycopene every day. Dosage may vary depending on physiological or pathological conditions. Lycopene up to 100 mg/day hasn't shown a side effect, in clinical studies. In animal studies, even 200 mg/kg didn't show any side effects either[1]. One side effect of lycopene noted in humans is lycopenaemia, reddish discoloration of the body, upon excessive lycopene consumption daily which retracted soon after the lycopene-rich diet was withdrawn.[9] Papaya raw fruit showed 2-9 times higher bioavailability than raw carrots and tomatoes.[5] Watermelon juice increased lycopene levels in postmenopausal women 3 fold.[6]

6) Caution: Lycopene is mostly embedded in the food matrix and is also heat-labile. Use the heat to break down the food matrix and avoiding heat mediated lycopene degradation, to increase the lycopene bioavailability.[2]

EVIDENCE: These compounds have been deduced from the MARK-AGE project, and alone they could be enough to deduce an anti-aging diet. But if there is evidence regarding mentioned methods, attenuation for biomarkers and antioxidants supplements, have some effect on decreasing aging, against COVID 19, or risk factors of

COVID 19, then it could be possible to allow dietary uptake of these against COVID19.

Earlier conclusion, complementary factors for the better metabolic utilization of lycopene in the body was proved in multiple research paper. Also, lycopene interaction with active compounds is crucial for obtaining optimum function in human health, and some beneficial actions may be a function of its isomers or metabolites. [1–4] Recently, a descriptive paper containing the lycopene mechanism against COVID 19 was also published.

1. Petyaev IM. Lycopene Deficiency in Ageing and Cardiovascular Disease. *Oxidative Medicine and Cellular Longevity*. 2016;2016. doi:10.1155/2016/3218605

2. Kong KW, Khoo HE, Prasad KN, Ismail A, Tan CP, Rajab NF. Revealing the power of the natural red pigment lycopene. *Molecules*. 2010;15(2):959-987. doi:10.3390/molecules15020959

3. Fielding JM, Rowley KG, Cooper P, O'Dea K. Increases in plasma lycopene concentration after consumption of tomatoes cooked with olive oil. *Asia Pacific Journal of Clinical Nutrition*. 2005;14(2):131-136. Accessed October 26, 2020. https://europepmc.org/article/med/15927929

4. Devaraj S, Mathur S, Basu A, et al. A Dose-Response Study on the Effects of Purified Lycopene Supplementation on Biomarkers of Oxidative Stress. *Journal of the American College of Nutrition*. 2008;27(2):267-273.

doi:10.1080/07315724.2008.10719699

5. Schweiggert RM, Kopec RE, Villalobos-Gutierrez MG, et al. Carotenoids are more bioavailable from papaya than from tomato and carrot in humans: A randomised cross-over study. *British Journal of Nutrition*. 2014;111(3):490-498. doi:10.1017/S0007114513002596

6. Ellis AC, Dudenbostel T, Crowe-White K. Watermelon Juice: a Novel Functional Food to Increase Circulating Lycopene in Older Adult Women. *Plant Foods for Human Nutrition*. 2019;74(2):200-203. doi:10.1007/s11130-019-00719-9

7. Yu J, Gleize B, Zhang L, Caris-Veyrat C, Renard CMGC. Heating tomato puree in the presence of lipids and onion: The impact of onion on lycopene isomerization. *Food Chemistry*. 2019;296:9-16. doi:10.1016/j.foodchem.2019.05.188

8. Böhm F, Edge R, Burke M, Truscott TG. Dietary uptake of lycopene protects human cells from singlet oxygen and nitrogen dioxide - ROS components from cigarette smoke. *Journal of Photochemistry and Photobiology B: Biology*. 2001;64(2-3):176-178. doi:10.1016/S1011-1344(01)00221-4

9. Caroselli C, Bruno G, Manara F. A rare cutaneous case of carotenosis cutis: Lycopenaemia. *Annals of Nutrition and Metabolism*. 2008;51(6):571-573. doi:10.1159/000114212

Chapter 5: Cysteine

CYSTEINE: a semi-essential amino acid, supplementary as N-acetyl cysteine (NAC), decreases peroxynitrite production in alveolar macrophages in lung pathologies.[1] A therapeutic intervention of NAC has been described for COVID 19 disease.[2] NAC is a well-tolerated mucolytic and boosts glutathione levels, which is involved in an endogenous antioxidant system exhibiting anti-aging properties,[3] and also documented for use against COVID 19.[4-6] Interestingly, Selenium is needed for optimal glutathione activity.[7,8] Selenium is also effective in COVID 19.[9] Vitamin B complex deficiency is harmful to COVID 19 patients.[9] Vitamin B6, B9, and B12 deficiency impair cysteine metabolism, and they together with Vitamin C show attenuation of methionine toxicity. Cysteine levels are increased by methionine consumption.[4,5] but methionine toxicity show death on 10 fold consumption and morbidity at 5 fold.[10]

Cysteine is found in animal and cereal proteins (beef, egg, whole grains).[11]

Diet and Dosage:

a) very small amounts of food items rich in methionine throughout day[4,5], and food items containing vitamin C, B6, B9, and B12 levels once daily:[10]
b) Low dose intermittent cysteine-rich food products throughout the day on alternate days.
c) High-dose single cysteine-rich meal.

Caution: Higher cysteine levels cause cysteine kidney stones, prevented by maintaining urine alkalization and good hydration through citrus juice and mineral water respectively.[12] Regular consumption of Cysteine may cause inhibition of in vivo cysteine synthesis.

1. Failli P, Palmieri L, D'Alfonso C, et al. Effect of N-acetyl-L-cysteine on peroxynitrite and superoxide anion production of lung alveolar macrophages in systemic sclerosis. *Nitric Oxide - Biology and Chemistry*. 2002;7(4):277-282. doi:10.1016/S1089-8603(02)00120-9

2. Poe FL, Corn J. N-Acetylcysteine: A potential therapeutic agent for SARS-CoV-2. *Medical Hypotheses*. 2020;143:109862. doi:10.1016/j.mehy.2020.109862

3. Mokhtari V, Afsharian P, Shahhoseini M, Kalantar SM, Moini A. A review on various uses of N-acetyl cysteine. *Cell Journal*. 2017;19(1):11-17. doi:10.22074/cellj.2016.4872

4. Clemente Plaza N, Reig García-Galbis M, Martínez-Espinosa RM. Effects of the Usage of l-Cysteine (l-Cys) on Human Health. *Molecules (Basel, Switzerland)*. 2018;23(3). doi:10.3390/molecules23030575

5. Yin J, Ren W, Yang G, et al. l-Cysteine metabolism and its nutritional implications. *Molecular Nutrition and Food Research*. 2016;60(1):134-146. doi:10.1002/mnfr.201500031

6. Guloyan V, Oganesian B, Baghdasaryan N, et al.

Glutathione supplementation as an adjunctive therapy in COVID-19. *Antioxidants*. 2020;9(10):1-22. doi:10.3390/antiox9100914

7. Somannavar MS, Kodliwadmath M V. Correlation between oxidative stress and antioxidant defence in south Indian urban vegetarians and non-vegetarians. *European Review for Medical and Pharmacological Sciences*. 2012;16(3):351-354.

8. Schomburg L. Dietary selenium and human health. *Nutrients*. 2017;9(1):22. doi:10.3390/nu9010022

9. Jayawardena R, Sooriyaarachchi P, Chourdakis M, Jeewandara C, Ranasinghe P. Enhancing immunity in viral infections, with special emphasis on COVID-19: A review. *Diabetes and Metabolic Syndrome: Clinical Research and Reviews*. 2020;14(4):367-382. doi:10.1016/j.dsx.2020.04.015

10. Garlick PJ. Toxicity of methionine in humans. *Journal of Nutrition*. 2006;136(6):1722S-1725S. doi:10.1093/jn/136.6.1722s

11. Larsson SC, Håkansson N, Wolk A. Dietary Cysteine and Other Amino Acids and Stroke Incidence in Women. *Stroke*. 2015;46(4):922-926. doi:10.1161/STROKEAHA.114.008022

12. Leslie SW, Nazzal L. Renal Calculi (Cystinuria, Cystine Stones). *StatPearls*. Published online January 21, 2018:1-6. Accessed October 30, 2020. http://www.ncbi.nlm.nih.gov/pubmed/29262245

Chapter 6: α TOCOPHEROL

α TOCOPHEROL (a supplementary form of Vitamin E): A well-known antioxidant, and used as a dietary supplement, and therapeutic administration. It is increased in GO and SGO. α-tocopherol supplementation lowers the dietary bioavailability of vitamin E, and α-tocopherol and γ-tocopherol levels are responsible for antioxidant and prooxidant action respectively,[1] thus indicating the composition of food sources while consuming vitamin E rich food should be considered. Second, vitamin E is a group of compounds, comprising tocopherols and tocotrienols. The supplementary form of vitamin E is α-tocopherol which shows toxicity at higher doses (>1000mg/day), but this toxicity is not observed with dietary vitamin E uptake. Further, tocotrienols show biological activities not shown by tocopherols. Synthetic and organic tocotrienols are structurally different and human receptors show stereospecificity, while there is no in vivo isomerization of these compounds. Thus, the dietary form of Vitamin E is superior to the supplementary form of vitamin E.[2,3] An increased uptake of Vitamin E-rich dietary sources, rich in α-tocopherol, and tocotrienols, and low in γ-tocopherol is recommended like olive oil, sunflower seeds, etc. Vitamin E supplementation has no protective effect and has been postulated as may be harmful in COVID 19.[4] But the mixed reports of benefits and harm, whether alpha-tocopherol or vitamin E as a whole, is in favor of the use of the dietary form of vitamin

E. Don't take tablets of α-tocopherol. Avoid food sources rich in γ-tocopherol and δ-tocopherol.[1]

1. Pizzino G, Irrera N, Cucinotta M, et al. Oxidative Stress: Harms and Benefits for Human Health. *Oxidative Medicine and Cellular Longevity*. 2017;2017. doi:10.1155/2017/8416763

2. Böhm V. Vitamin E. *Antioxidants*. 2018;7(3):44. doi:10.3390/ANTIOX7030044

3. Rizvi S, Raza ST, Ahmed F, Ahmad A, Abbas S, Mahdi F. The role of Vitamin E in human health and some diseases. *Sultan Qaboos University Medical Journal*. 2014;14(2):e157-e165. https://pubmed.ncbi.nlm.nih.gov/24790736

4. Jayawardena R, Sooriyaarachchi P, Chourdakis M, Jeewandara C, Ranasinghe P. Enhancing immunity in viral infections, with special emphasis on COVID-19: A review. *Diabetes and Metabolic Syndrome: Clinical Research and Reviews*. 2020;14(4):367-382. doi:10.1016/j.dsx.2020.04.015

Chapter 7: Malondialdehyde

Malondialdehyde (MDA): A biomarker of lipid peroxidation, and oxidative stress, is a reactive electrophile species; forming covalent protein adducts, Advanced Lipoxidation End-products (ALE), Advanced Glycation end products (AGE), and several types of mutagenic DNA adducts. High MDA level is seen in high fatty foods consumption and rancid food uptake, and low MDA level in high fruit and vegetable consumption.[1] Oral MDA supplementation increases plasma MDA levels. Approach to lower plasma MDA level:

1.) Decreasing MDA synthesis implies lowering lipid peroxidation, and it would refer to free radical scavengers, and reactive species scavengers, both ROS and RNS.[1-3]
2.) Increasing MDA excretion is easier as it is water-soluble,[1] increasing body water turnover.
3.) Decreasing MDA action can be done by taurine,[4] NAC, carnosine,[2] histamine,[5] and melatonin[2,6]. Among them, carnosine is better than NAC.[2]

Apart from dietary sources, regular exercise of moderate to severe intensity,[1] and pharmacological administration of folate supplementation and vitamin D3 supplementation has shown to decrease levels of malondialdehyde.[7-11] No direct link between vitamin D and COVID 19 severity was accounted for, but recent trials find it useful.[12] Taurine shows cytoprotective effect via induction of mitochondrial biogenesis, restoration of mitochondrial membrane potential, and partial restoration of NO generation.[4,13] Taurine reduces oxidative stress in diabetes,[14] and is protective in lung pathologies.[15,16] Carnosine protects against cross-linking by non-enzymatic Glycation, is helpful in neurodegenerative diseases, like Alzheimer's, which is also an age-related disease.[2,13] Melatonin helps maintain a circadian rhythm, removes unsaturated carbonyls, and protects against oxidative stress.[6,17] Histamine makes stable products with MDA,[5] but is associated with allergic reactions and food poisoning, so excluded. An account of carnosine,[18–20] and melatonin,[21,22] action against COVID 19 has been presented to some extent, and trials are underway for melatonin.[23] Interventions for different methods have been presented below

1) Decrease MDA synthesis:
   a) Decrease lipid peroxidation: via free radical, RNS, and ROS scavengers like Vitamin C (guava, kiwi, strawberry orange, tomato), Vitamin E, Carotenoids (carrot, spinach), other antioxidants like lycopene, quercetin, etc.
   b) Vitamin D supplementation: Fish, eggs, fortified food products.[8,9,11]
2) Increase MDA excretion: as MDA is water-soluble, it can be easily excreted if some supra-hydration is maintained. Simply drinking a liter of more water than every day will increase urine output and

enable MDA excretion. Or, maintaining adequate hydration before MDA-rich meal consumption.
3) Decrease MDA action:
   a) Carnosine is found in chicken breasts, beef (only in animal food sources, not found in plant food sources). It is water-soluble, boiling decreases carnosine level as released in water. Grilling or roasting is not advised as it increases MDA levels. Microwave heating is recommended; otherwise stewing is the second-best option, as the carnosine released in water can still be consumed.[24] Dosage: 8.66 mg/kg body weight per day (estimated). A detailed account of dosage is available for different conditions.[2,13]
   b) Taurine is found in animal food products.[14] Increased cysteine consumption increases taurine levels.[14,25] It is water-soluble, and on oral consumption, it peaks at 1-1.5 hours after oral administration, and is excreted via bile conjugation, has renal clearance, and returns to normal levels in 6 hours. Food intake delays absorption.[14,24,25] Boiling decreases taurine level in food, as it is released in water. Microwave heating is recommended; otherwise cooking by boiling is the second-best option, as taurine released in water can still be consumed as gravy.[24] Dosage: 1.07 mg/kg body weight per day (Estimated). A detailed account of dosage for different conditions is available.[4,13]

c) Melatonin is found in pistachios, mushrooms, aged/frozen berries, nuts, fruits, etc.[26] Tryptophan-rich food products increase melatonin levels[26]. It has poor oral bioavailability and is higher in females than male.[26]. Few studied instances of melatonin diet have been mentioned in the dietary form below
   (1) Pistachios
      (a) ½ to 1 serving 1-2 hours before bedtime with 2-3 pieces at a close interval of 8-10 hours in the daytime.[26]
      (b) 44gm (1 serving) of pistachios in the afternoon.[27]
   (2) Mushrooms or fruits should be added in breakfast and dinner for life, or at least in two meals per day 12 hours apart.[26,27]
  ii) Dose: 0.2 e 5 mg for adults close to bedtime. Dosage can be regulated by diet through subjective symptomatic assessment.[6,17] Upon consumption of higher dosage, next day sleepiness will be experienced requiring to lower the dose slightly.
  iii) Caution: Higher levels of melatonin induce sleepiness, so should be taken in moderate amount in the nighttime, 1-2 hours before bed.[17]
d) Cysteine (discussed under cysteine heading)

4) Behavioral approaches affecting MDA
   a) High fruits and vegetable consumption.[1,28]
   b) Exercising regularly, at medium to severe intensity lowers MDA levels.[1]
   c) Eat food hot: Oral administration of MDA has a deleterious effect, so avoiding rancid food which has higher MDA levels is a good and simple approach to maintain lower MDA levels.
   d) Smoking cessation, as smoking individuals have higher MDA levels.[1,29]
   e) Refrigerated animal meats show higher MDA levels.[24]
   f) MDA is present in higher amounts in animal food products, but major attenuating factors taurine, carnosine, histamine, and melatonin, are also present in higher amounts in animal food products. Boiling and then grilling meat showed the highest increase in MDA levels in animal meat. Thus, presenting a cuisine that keeps MDA uptake low and its attenuating factors high, in animal food products is a question of testing permutations and combinations of different meals. From currently available data, cooking by boiling to make gravy for consumption is the best available cuisine.[24]

1. Saieva C, Peluso M, Palli D, et al. Dietary and lifestyle determinants of malondialdehyde DNA adducts in a representative sample of the Florence

City population. *Mutagenesis*. 2016;31(4):475-480. doi:10.1093/mutage/gew012

2. Cheng J, Wang F, Yu DF, Wu PF, Chen JG. The cytotoxic mechanism of malondialdehyde and protective effect of carnosine via protein cross-linking/mitochondrial dysfunction/reactive oxygen species/MAPK pathway in neurons. *European Journal of Pharmacology*. 2011;650(1):184-194. doi:10.1016/j.ejphar.2010.09.033

3. Somannavar MS, Kodliwadmath M V. Correlation between oxidative stress and antioxidant defence in south Indian urban vegetarians and non-vegetarians. *European Review for Medical and Pharmacological Sciences*. 2012;16(3):351-354.

4. Cai JG, Luo LM, Tang H, Zhou L. Cytotoxicity of Malondialdehyde and Cytoprotective Effects of Taurine via Oxidative Stress and PGC-1α Signal Pathway in C2C12 Cells. *Molecular Biology*. 2018;52(4):532-542. doi:10.1134/S0026898418040043

5. Li L, Li G, Sheng S, Yin D. Substantial reaction between histamine and malondialdehyde: A new observation of carbonyl stress. *Neuroendocrinology Letters*. 2005;26(6):799-805.

6. Tordjman S, Chokron S, Delorme R, et al. Melatonin: Pharmacology, Functions and Therapeutic Benefits. *Current Neuropharmacology*. 2017;15(3):434-443. doi:10.2174/1570159x14666161228122115

7. Aghamohammadi V, Gargari BP, Aliasgharzadeh A. Effect of Folic Acid Supplementation on

Homocysteine, Serum Total Antioxidant Capacity, and Malondialdehyde in Patients with Type 2 Diabetes Mellitus. *Journal of the American College of Nutrition*. 2011;30(3):210-215. doi:10.1080/07315724.2011.10719962

8. Bahrami LS, Sezavar Seyedi Jandaghi SH, Janani L, et al. Vitamin D supplementation and serum heat shock protein 60 levels in patients with coronary heart disease: A randomized clinical trial. *Nutrition and Metabolism*. 2018;15(1):56. doi:10.1186/s12986-018-0292-9

9. Gu JW, Liu JH, Xiao HN, et al. Relationship between plasma levels of 25-hydroxyvitamin D and arterial stiffness in elderly Chinese with non-dipper hypertension: An observational study. *Medicine (United States)*. 2020;99(7):e19200-e19200. doi:10.1097/MD.0000000000019200

10. Caroselli C, Bruno G, Manara F. A rare cutaneous case of carotenosis cutis: Lycopenaemia. *Annals of Nutrition and Metabolism*. 2008;51(6):571-573. doi:10.1159/000114212

11. Ahmad A, Singhal U, Hossain MM, Islam N, Rizvi I. The role of the endogenous antioxidant enzymes and malondialdehyde in essential hypertension. *Journal of Clinical and Diagnostic Research*. 2013;7(6):987-990. doi:10.7860/JCDR/2013/5829.3091

12. Hernández JL, Nan D, Fernandez-Ayala M, et al. Vitamin D Status in Hospitalized Patients With SARS-CoV-2 Infection. *The Journal of Clinical Endocrinology & Metabolism*. Published online

October 27, 2020. doi:10.1210/clinem/dgaa733

13. Wu G. *Important Roles of Dietary Taurine, Creatine, Carnosine, Anserine and 4-Hydroxyproline in Human Nutrition and Health*. Vol 52. Springer Vienna; 2020. doi:10.1007/s00726-020-02823-6

14. Maleki V, Mahdavi R, Hajizadeh-Sharafabad F, Alizadeh M. The effects of taurine supplementation on oxidative stress indices and inflammation biomarkers in patients with type 2 diabetes: A randomized, double-blind, placebo-controlled trial. *Diabetology and Metabolic Syndrome*. 2020;12(1):9. doi:10.1186/s13098-020-0518-7

15. Bernatchez JA, McCall LI. Insights gained into respiratory infection pathogenesis using lung tissue metabolomics. *PLoS Pathogens*. 2020;16(7):e1008662-e1008662. doi:10.1371/journal.ppat.1008662

16. Thomas T, Stefanoni D, Reisz JA, et al. COVID-19 infection alters kynurenine and fatty acid metabolism, correlating with IL-6 levels and renal status. *JCI Insight*. 2020;5(14):e140327. doi:10.1172/JCI.INSIGHT.140327

17. Pereira N, Naufel MF, Ribeiro EB, Tufik S, Hachul H. Influence of Dietary Sources of Melatonin on Sleep Quality: A Review. *Journal of Food Science*. 2020;85(1):5-13. doi:10.1111/1750-3841.14952

18. Hipkiss AR. COVID-19 and senotherapeutics: Any role for the naturally-occurring dipeptide carnosine? *Aging and Disease*. 2020;11(4):737-741. doi:10.14336/AD.2020.0518

19. Lopachev A V., Kazanskaya RB, Khutorova A V., Fedorova TN. An overview of the pathogenic mechanisms involved in severe cases of COVID-19 infection, and the proposal of salicyl-carnosine as a potential drug for its treatment. *European Journal of Pharmacology*. 2020;886:173457. doi:10.1016/j.ejphar.2020.173457

20. Jindal C, Kumar S, Sharma S, Choi YM, Efird JT. The prevention and management of covid-19: Seeking a practical and timely solution. *International Journal of Environmental Research and Public Health*. 2020;17(11):3986. doi:10.3390/ijerph17113986

21. Bahrampour Juybari K, Pourhanifeh MH, Hosseinzadeh A, Hemati K, Mehrzadi S. Melatonin potentials against viral infections including COVID-19: Current evidence and new findings. *Virus Research*. 2020;287:198108. doi:10.1016/j.virusres.2020.198108

22. Zhang R, Wang X, Ni L, et al. COVID-19: Melatonin as a potential adjuvant treatment. *Life Sciences*. 2020;250:117583. doi:10.1016/j.lfs.2020.117583

23. Nct. Melatonin Agonist on Hospitalized Patients With Confirmed or Suspected COVID-19. *https://clinicaltrials.gov/show/NCT04470297*. Published online 2020. https://www.cochranelibrary.com/central/doi/10.1002/central/CN-02134434/full

24. Okolie NP, Okugbo OT. a Comparative Study of Malondialdehyde Contents of Some Meat and Fish Samples Processed By Different Methods. *Journal of Pharmaceutical and Scientific Innovation*.

2013;2(4):26-29. doi:10.7897/2277-4572.02448

25. Mokhtari V, Afsharian P, Shahhoseini M, Kalantar SM, Moini A. A review on various uses of N-acetyl cysteine. *Cell Journal*. 2017;19(1):11-17. doi:10.22074/cellj.2016.4872

26. Meng X, Li Y, Li S, et al. Dietary sources and bioactivities of melatonin. *Nutrients*. 2017;9(4):367. doi:10.3390/nu9040367

27. Fantino M, Bichard C, Mistretta F, Bellisle F. Daily consumption of pistachios over 12 weeks improves dietary profile without increasing body weight in healthy women: A randomized controlled intervention. *Appetite*. 2020;144:104483. doi:10.1016/j.appet.2019.104483

28. Peluso M, Munnia A, Piro S, et al. Fruit and vegetable and fried food consumption and 3-(2-deoxy-β-D- erythro-pentafuranosyl)pyrimido[1,2-α] purin-10(3H)-one deoxyguanosine adduct formation. *Free Radical Research*. 2012;46(1):85-92. doi:10.3109/10715762.2011.640676

29. Shah AA, Khand F, Khand TU. Effect of smoking on serum xanthine oxidase, malondialdehyde, ascorbic acid and α-tocopherol levels in healthy male subjects. *Pakistan Journal of Medical Sciences*. 2015;31(1):146-149. doi:10.12669/pjms.311.6148

Chapter 8: 3-Nitro tyrosine

3- Nitro tyrosine (3NT): Increased only in GO, and not SGO, thus a genetic adaptation. It is a product of tyrosine nitration, mediated by peroxynitrite dependent, peroxynitrite independent, and free radical-mediated pathways. Thus, an increased serum level is either more tyrosine nitration, via any tyrosine nitration pathway; or decreased 3-nitro tyrosine catabolism. The major contribution is by peroxynitrite alone. In the entire mechanism of 3NT, including action, formation, and elimination, only tyrosine radical formation is associated with multiple essential benefits.[1,2] Dietary elements changing 3NT levels in favor of process has been postulated by referencing available methods:

1) Peroxynitrite dependent-
    a) N-acetyl-cysteine decreases peroxynitrite formation.[3]
    b) Herbs: Choi et al, showed peroxynitrite scavenging potency of different herbs; Witch hazel bark, rosemary, jasmine tea, sage, slippery elm, black walnut leaf, Queen Anne's lace, and Linden flower. Choi et al, also found Hamamelitannin, as a major active component of witch hazel bark with strong peroxynitrite scavenging.[4]
    c) Vitamin C: water-soluble, highly bioavailable, gives extracellular protection against peroxynitrite.[5] Citrus family fruits like kiwi, amla, orange, and

vegetables such as broccoli, tomatoes, and peppers are rich in vitamin C.[6]

d) Quercetin: lipid-soluble, show intracellular protection against peroxynitrite.[5] Found in red onion, grapes, blueberries, cherries, apples, and broccoli.[7] Its bioavailability can be increased by adding vitamin C, consuming along with non-digestible fibers, or breaking the food matrix. Taking up with dietary fat helps in absorption.[8]

e) (−)-epigallocatechin gallate: best-known inhibitor of peroxynitrite meditated tyrosine nitration.[9] Found in green tea, cocoa.[7,10]

2) Protection against peroxynitrite independent enzymatic peroxide action:
   a) Glutathione endogenous production is increased by NAC, α-lipoic acid, raw liver, whey protein, or milk thistle.[11–13]
   b) Selenium: Brazilian nuts, eggs, and chicken are major sources. However, caution should be taken against selenium toxicity and deficiency.[14]

3) Free radical scavengers for decreasing free radical/heavy metal transitional state mediated 3NT formation.[1]

Vitamin C, at high intravenous doses, shows rapid recovery in critically ill COVID 19 patients,[15], and maybe beneficial in COVID 19 infection.[16] Quercetin reduces virus-host interaction of COVID 19 with ACE-2, and has been identified with senolytic properties, and was found to be potentially effective against COVID19 disease.[17] NAC, glutathione, and selenium have already been discussed under the cysteine heading. Meals have been suggested based on available research materials:

1) For peroxynitrite mediated:
   a) Vitamin C with Quercetin: it is recommended to consume vitamin C pre-meal and quercetin during or after the meal.
      i) Vitamin C: 5-9 servings of fresh citrus fruits or animal sources like animal liver. [6]
      ii) Quercetin is lipophilic, so together would be good for extracellular and intracellular scavenging, respectively[5,8]. Break down the food matrix or decrease its size as much as you can, maybe using a shredder, and increase the use of quercetin-rich food in regular meals. Use oil to incorporate, or simply incorporate it into meals.[8]
   b) (−)-epigallocatechin gallate:
      i) 2-3 cups of green tea a day prepared by brewing at 100 °C for 9.50 min with water/tea concentration 70.0 mL/g, and 230 μm gives the highest antioxidant property[18]. So try to approach as close as possible;
      ii) consume cocoa (raw dark chocolates).[7]
      iii) N acetylcysteine: discussed below
2) Peroxide scavengers
   a) Glutathione: NAC is preferred, but a spike in glutathione levels is followed by rapid decline, so

regular uptake in small dosages throughout the day.[19]

b) Selenium: Brazilian nuts, fish, eggs, fortified food consumption.[14]

1. Campolo N, Issoglio FM, Estrin DA, Bartesaghi S, Radi R. 3-Nitrotyrosine and related derivatives in proteins: precursors, radical intermediates and impact in function. *Essays in Biochemistry*. 2020;64(1):111-133. doi:10.1042/ebc20190052

2. Weber D, Stuetz W, Toussaint O, et al. Associations between Specific Redox Biomarkers and Age in a Large European Cohort: The MARK-AGE Project. *Oxidative Medicine and Cellular Longevity*. 2017;2017. doi:10.1155/2017/1401452

3. Failli P, Palmieri L, D'Alfonso C, et al. Effect of N-acetyl-L-cysteine on peroxynitrite and superoxide anion production of lung alveolar macrophages in systemic sclerosis. *Nitric Oxide - Biology and Chemistry*. 2002;7(4):277-282. doi:10.1016/S1089-8603(02)00120-9

4. Choi HR, Choi JS, Han YN, Bae SJ, Chung HY. Peroxynitrite scavenging activity of herb extracts. *Phytotherapy Research*. 2002;16(4):364-367. doi:10.1002/ptr.904

5. Balavoine GGA, Geletii Y V. Peroxynitrite scavenging by different antioxidants. Part I: Convenient assay. *Nitric Oxide - Biology and Chemistry*. 1999;3(1):40-54. doi:10.1006/niox.1999.0206

6. Lykkesfeldt J, Michels AJ, Frei B. Vitamin C.

Advances in Nutrition. 2014;5(1):16-18. doi:10.3945/an.113.005157

7. Si H, Liu D. Dietary antiaging phytochemicals and mechanisms associated with prolonged survival. *Journal of Nutritional Biochemistry.* 2014;25(6):581-591. doi:10.1016/j.jnutbio.2014.02.001

8. Guo Y, Bruno RS. Endogenous and exogenous mediators of quercetin bioavailability. *Journal of Nutritional Biochemistry.* 2015;26(3):201-210. doi:10.1016/j.jnutbio.2014.10.008

9. Fiala FS, Sodum RS, Bhattacharya M, Li H. (-)-Epigallocatechin gallate, a polyphenolic tea antioxidant, inhibits peroxynitrite-mediated formation of 8-oxodeoxyguanosine and 3-nitrotyrosine. *Experientia.* 1996;52(9):922-926. doi:10.1007/BF01938881

10. Suzuki Y, Miyoshi N, Isemura M. Health-promoting effects of green tea. *Proceedings of the Japan Academy Series B: Physical and Biological Sciences.* 2012;88(3):88-101. doi:10.2183/pjab.88.88

11. Somannavar MS, Kodliwadmath M V. Correlation between oxidative stress and antioxidant defence in south Indian urban vegetarians and non-vegetarians. *European Review for Medical and Pharmacological Sciences.* 2012;16(3):351-354.

12. Ahmad A, Singhal U, Hossain MM, Islam N, Rizvi I. The role of the endogenous antioxidant enzymes and malondialdehyde in essential hypertension. *Journal of Clinical and Diagnostic Research.* 2013;7(6):987-990.

doi:10.7860/JCDR/2013/5829.3091

13. Mokhtari V, Afsharian P, Shahhoseini M, Kalantar SM, Moini A. A review on various uses of N-acetyl cysteine. *Cell Journal*. 2017;19(1):11-17. doi:10.22074/cellj.2016.4872

14. Schomburg L. Dietary selenium and human health. *Nutrients*. 2017;9(1):22. doi:10.3390/nu9010022

15. Khan HMW, Parikh N, Megala SM, Predeteanu GS. Unusual early recovery of a critical COVID-19 patient after administration of intravenous vitamin C. *American Journal of Case Reports*. 2020;21:1-6. doi:10.12659/AJCR.925521

16. Jayawardena R, Sooriyaarachchi P, Chourdakis M, Jeewandara C, Ranasinghe P. Enhancing immunity in viral infections, with special emphasis on COVID-19: A review. *Diabetes and Metabolic Syndrome: Clinical Research and Reviews*. 2020;14(4):367-382. doi:10.1016/j.dsx.2020.04.015

17. Sargiacomo C, Sotgia F, Lisanti MP. COVID-19 and chronological aging: Senolytics and other anti-aging drugs for the treatment or prevention of corona virus infection? *Aging*. 2020;12(8):6511-6517. doi:10.18632/AGING.103001

18. Liu Y, Luo L, Liao C, Chen L, Wang J, Zeng L. Effects of brewing conditions on the phytochemical composition, sensory qualities and antioxidant activity of green tea infusion: A study using response surface methodology. *Food Chemistry*. 2018;269:24-34. doi:10.1016/j.foodchem.2018.06.130

19. Clemente Plaza N, Reig García-Galbis M, Martínez-Espinosa RM. Effects of the Usage of l-Cysteine (l-Cys) on Human Health. *Molecules (Basel, Switzerland)*. 2018;23(3). doi:10.3390/molecules23030575

Chapter 9: Resveratrol

A HYPOTHETICAL CHALLENGE

Navigation through the previous-mentioned biomarkers may stress individual cells under less oxidative damage and decreased residual cellular garbage (DNA adducts, AGEPs, ALEPs, etc.). In such cellular instances, cells can approach their full potential, and it may increase vulnerability to hypersensitivity reactions, or diet toxicity-induced metabolic alterations, as seen in methionine toxicity.[1,2] To maintain and avoid such challenge, naturally occurring phytochemical especially Resveratrol is useful,[2] and is a part of UDAT. Curcumin also exerts a similar effect but appears less effective than resveratrol.[2] Resveratrol is found in red wine, grapes, apple, peanut, soy, berries[3]. It has extremely low bioavailability,[3] and is impossible to eat enough to reach therapeutic concentration.[4] However, resveratrol and its derivatives differ in potency, and the hydrophobic nature of resveratrol, allows normal doses for longer durations to elicit benefits.[4] Few recommendations based on research are given:

1) A single serving of grapes, preferably after the meal (preferably dinner).[4]
2) A single serving of red wine.[3]
3) Apple, peanuts, soy, or others in amount as desired.

Drug interaction should be cautioned for resveratrol.[2] To avoid this either consult your doctor or refer to 'drug interaction checker' yourself on Medscape on the following link: https://reference.medscape.com/drug-interactionchecker.

1. Garlick PJ. Toxicity of methionine in humans. *Journal of Nutrition*. 2006;136(6):1722S-1725S. doi:10.1093/jn/136.6.1722s

2. Si H, Liu D. Dietary antiaging phytochemicals and mechanisms associated with prolonged survival. *Journal of Nutritional Biochemistry*. 2014;25(6):581-591. doi:10.1016/j.jnutbio.2014.02.001

3. Weiskirchen S, Weiskirchen R. Resveratrol: How Much Wine Do You Have to Drink to Stay Healthy? *Advances in nutrition (Bethesda, Md)*. 2016;7(4):706-718. doi:10.3945/an.115.011627

4. Salehi B, Mishra AP, Nigam M, et al. Resveratrol: A Double-Edged Sword in Health Benefits. *Biomedicines*. 2018;6(3):91. doi:10.3390/biomedicines6030091

Chapter 10: UDAT

There is an effect of diet and cuisine, which can elicit the anti-aging properties of multiple food products. And here a dietary plan has been presented. The principles applied are more important than the diet indicated. As there is a variation of food products in different areas, it is recommended to understand the principle and seek the help of a health professional in crafting area-wise economical diet. So this is going to be the foundational basis of Universal Dietary Adjunct Therapy (UDAT). This dietary method when combined with existing norms of micronutrients and macronutrients, one may call it, Universal Dietary Therapy. As an attempt from Mark-Age Project,[1,2] here is a reference to formulated diet, UDAT. I haven't gone into details, of any other disease, other than COVID19, but here approaching synchronization with aging, and maybe avoiding or delaying the age-expected deterioration, should have the upper hand in achieving better health. Deductions are unethical in medical science. But, the reasons for holding clinical trials are important to understand pharmacokinetics, safety levels, side effects, and rare complications. However, these food products are present in the community for quite a long time. And their side effects are known, and well understood, and have higher margins of safety levels, even clinically proven.[3,4,13–16,5–12]

One major limitation on the very fundamental of research study, population and geographical uniformity is questionable. MARK-AGE was conducted on the European population. However, the redox markers are directed at the genetic level and the genetic resemblance of the entire human population is more than significant, higher than 99.9%. But, if the question has to be scientifically answered, conduct an identical mark-age project structured research for different geographical/regional populations.

1. Bürkle A, Moreno-Villanueva M, Bernhard J, et al. MARK-AGE biomarkers of ageing. *Mechanisms of Ageing and Development*. 2015;151:2-12. doi:10.1016/j.mad.2015.03.006

2. Weber D, Stuetz W, Toussaint O, et al. Associations between Specific Redox Biomarkers and Age in a Large European Cohort: The MARK-AGE Project. *Oxidative Medicine and Cellular Longevity*. 2017;2017. doi:10.1155/2017/1401452

3. Salehi B, Mishra AP, Nigam M, et al. Resveratrol: A Double-Edged Sword in Health Benefits. *Biomedicines*. 2018;6(3):91. doi:10.3390/biomedicines6030091

4. Fielding JM, Rowley KG, Cooper P, O'Dea K. Increases in plasma lycopene concentration after consumption of tomatoes cooked with olive oil. *Asia Pacific Journal of Clinical Nutrition*. 2005;14(2):131-136. Accessed October 26, 2020. https://europepmc.org/article/med/15927929

5. Sameem B, Khan F, Niaz K. l-Cysteine. Published online 2019:53-58.

doi:https://doi.org/10.1016/B978-0-12-812491-8.00007-2

6. Guo Y, Bruno RS. Endogenous and exogenous mediators of quercetin bioavailability. *Journal of Nutritional Biochemistry*. 2015;26(3):201-210. doi:10.1016/j.jnutbio.2014.10.008

7. Liu Y, Luo L, Liao C, Chen L, Wang J, Zeng L. Effects of brewing conditions on the phytochemical composition, sensory qualities and antioxidant activity of green tea infusion: A study using response surface methodology. *Food Chemistry*. 2018;269:24-34. doi:10.1016/j.foodchem.2018.06.130

8. Wu G. *Important Roles of Dietary Taurine, Creatine, Carnosine, Anserine and 4-Hydroxyproline in Human Nutrition and Health*. Vol 52. Springer Vienna; 2020. doi:10.1007/s00726-020-02823-6

9. Rizvi S, Raza ST, Ahmed F, Ahmad A, Abbas S, Mahdi F. The role of Vitamin E in human health and some diseases. *Sultan Qaboos University Medical Journal*. 2014;14(2):e157-e165. https://pubmed.ncbi.nlm.nih.gov/24790736

10. Schomburg L. Dietary selenium and human health. *Nutrients*. 2017;9(1):22. doi:10.3390/nu9010022

11. Jayawardena R, Sooriyaarachchi P, Chourdakis M, Jeewandara C, Ranasinghe P. Enhancing immunity in viral infections, with special emphasis on COVID-19: A review. *Diabetes and Metabolic Syndrome: Clinical Research and Reviews*. 2020;14(4):367-382. doi:10.1016/j.dsx.2020.04.015

12. Böhm V. Vitamin E. *Antioxidants*. 2018;7(3):44. doi:10.3390/ANTIOX7030044

13. Lykkesfeldt J, Michels AJ, Frei B. Vitamin C. *Advances in Nutrition*. 2014;5(1):16-18. doi:10.3945/an.113.005157

14. Devaraj S, Mathur S, Basu A, et al. A Dose-Response Study on the Effects of Purified Lycopene Supplementation on Biomarkers of Oxidative Stress. *Journal of the American College of Nutrition*. 2008;27(2):267-273. doi:10.1080/07315724.2008.10719699

15. Garlick PJ. Toxicity of methionine in humans. *Journal of Nutrition*. 2006;136(6):1722S-1725S. doi:10.1093/jn/136.6.1722s

16. Meng X, Li Y, Li S, et al. Dietary sources and bioactivities of melatonin. *Nutrients*. 2017;9(4):367. doi:10.3390/nu9040367

SUMMARY: UDAT CHART

	BIOMARKERS/ ANTIOXIDANTS	PRINCIPLE	SUB-PRINCIPLE	APPROACH	FOOD SOURCES
1	LYCOPENE	Increasing lycopene levels along with supplements		Lycopene rich food sources	Watermelon[1], Tomato[2,3] carrot, papaya[4],
. .	..	..		Supplements that help lycopene metabolism	Vitamin C[2] quercetin, Vitamin E[5]
2.	3-nitrotyrosine	Peroxynitrite dependent[6]	Decrease Peroxynitrite formation	N acetylcysteine (cysteine)[7]	Animal and cereal proteins (beef, eggs, whole grains)[8,9]
. .	..	..	Protect against peroxynitrite	Quercetin	Elderberries, blueberries,

.	..	..			vitamin C	cherries, onions, apples, and broccoli[10]
.	..	..			vitamin C	guava, kiwi, strawberry orange, tomato[11]
.	..	..			EPCG	Green tea[10]
.	..	..			EPCG	Vitamin C (guava, kiwi, strawberry orange, tomato)
.	..		Peroxynitrite independent[6]	Free radical scavenging	Free radical scavengers	Vitamin E, Carotenoids (carrot, spinach), other antioxidants
.	..	..		Protection against peroxynitrite independent	Glutathione	NAC, VIT C, VIT B, selenium-rich food sources[12].

#						
					enzymatic peroxide action	
.	..	..	..		Selenium[13]	Brazilian nut, spinach, egg
.	..	..	..	Free radical/ heavy metal transitional state mediated[6]	Free radical scavenging	Free radical scavenger	Vitamin C (guava, kiwi, strawberry orange, tomato) Vitamin E, Carotenoids (carrot, spinach), other antioxidants
3.	Cysteine			Increase cysteine levels		Increase methionine consumption with vitamin B6, B12, B9, and C[9,14]	Methionine rich food sources (poultry, eggs, etc.), Vit B6, Vit B9, Vit B12, Vit C (all taken

#				
			Increase cysteine dietary sources	together) Animal and cereal proteins (beef, egg, whole grains)[8]
4.	α TOCOPHEROL	Increase vitamin E levels	Increase dietary consumption of high α tocopherol and low γ tocopherol.	Olive oil, sunflower seeds[15]
5.	Malondialdehyde	Decrease MDA synthesis	Decrease lipid peroxidation, via free radical, RNS, and ROS scavengers[16]	Vitamin C (guava, kiwi, strawberry orange, tomato) Vitamin E, Carotenoids (carrot, spinach), other antioxida

· ·	· ·	· ·		Vitamin D[17]	nts[16]. Fish, eggs, fortified food products
· ·	· ·	Increase MDA excretion		Increasing water consumption	Drink water, one liter more than you do, or maintain hydration.
· ·	· ·	Decrease MDA action		Carnosine[18]	Chicken breasts[19]
· ·	· ·			Melatonin	Pistachios, mushroom, nuts, fruits and vegetables[20], milk[21]
· ·	· ·			NAC	Poultry, egg, whole grains, sunflower seeds[22]
· ·	· ·			Taurine[2]	Meat,

·			fish, dairy products.[3]
· ·	··	··	··	Cysteine-rich food products- Animal and cereal proteins (beef, eggs, whole grains)[8,9]
· ·	··	Behavioral approaches	Decreased MDA plasma levels	High fruit and vegetable content in diet[24]. Regular exercise of medium/severe intensity[25]
· ·	··	··	··	
· ·	··	··	··	Avoiding rancid food (eat food hot, or refrigerate)

					smoking cessation[25]
6.	Resveratrol	Avoid uncontrolled reactions		Avoid alteration in metabolic pathways	Red wine, grapes[10]

Table I SUMMARY

1. Ellis AC, Dudenbostel T, Crowe-White K. Watermelon Juice: a Novel Functional Food to Increase Circulating Lycopene in Older Adult Women. *Plant Foods for Human Nutrition*. 2019;74(2):200-203. doi:10.1007/s11130-019-00719-9

2. Böhm F, Edge R, Burke M, Truscott TG. Dietary uptake of lycopene protects human cells from singlet oxygen and nitrogen dioxide - ROS components from cigarette smoke. *Journal of Photochemistry and Photobiology B: Biology*. 2001;64(2-3):176-178. doi:10.1016/S1011-1344(01)00221-4

3. Devaraj S, Mathur S, Basu A, et al. A Dose-Response Study on the Effects of Purified Lycopene Supplementation on Biomarkers of Oxidative Stress. *Journal of the American College of Nutrition*. 2008;27(2):267-273. doi:10.1080/07315724.2008.10719699

4. Schweiggert RM, Kopec RE, Villalobos-Gutierrez MG,

et al. Carotenoids are more bioavailable from papaya than from tomato and carrot in humans: A randomised cross-over study. *British Journal of Nutrition*. 2014;111(3):490-498. doi:10.1017/S0007114513002596

5. Kong KW, Khoo HE, Prasad KN, Ismail A, Tan CP, Rajab NF. Revealing the power of the natural red pigment lycopene. *Molecules*. 2010;15(2):959-987. doi:10.3390/molecules15020959

6. Campolo N, Issoglio FM, Estrin DA, Bartesaghi S, Radi R. 3-Nitrotyrosine and related derivatives in proteins: precursors, radical intermediates and impact in function. *Essays in Biochemistry*. 2020;64(1):111-133. doi:10.1042/ebc20190052

7. Failli P, Palmieri L, D'Alfonso C, et al. Effect of N-acetyl-L-cysteine on peroxynitrite and superoxide anion production of lung alveolar macrophages in systemic sclerosis. *Nitric Oxide - Biology and Chemistry*. 2002;7(4):277-282. doi:10.1016/S1089-8603(02)00120-9

8. Larsson SC, Håkansson N, Wolk A. Dietary Cysteine and Other Amino Acids and Stroke Incidence in Women. *Stroke*. 2015;46(4):922-926. doi:10.1161/STROKEAHA.114.008022

9. Yin J, Ren W, Yang G, et al. l-Cysteine metabolism and its nutritional implications. *Molecular Nutrition and Food Research*. 2016;60(1):134-146. doi:10.1002/mnfr.201500031

10. Si H, Liu D. Dietary antiaging phytochemicals and mechanisms associated with prolonged survival.

Journal of Nutritional Biochemistry. 2014;25(6):581-591. doi:10.1016/j.jnutbio.2014.02.001

11. Lykkesfeldt J, Michels AJ, Frei B. Vitamin C. *Advances in Nutrition*. 2014;5(1):16-18. doi:10.3945/an.113.005157

12. Poe FL, Corn J. N-Acetylcysteine: A potential therapeutic agent for SARS-CoV-2. *Medical Hypotheses*. 2020;143:109862. doi:10.1016/j.mehy.2020.109862

13. Schomburg L. Dietary selenium and human health. *Nutrients*. 2017;9(1):22. doi:10.3390/nu9010022

14. Garlick PJ. Toxicity of methionine in humans. *Journal of Nutrition*. 2006;136(6):1722S-1725S. doi:10.1093/jn/136.6.1722s

15. Pizzino G, Irrera N, Cucinotta M, et al. Oxidative Stress: Harms and Benefits for Human Health. *Oxidative Medicine and Cellular Longevity*. 2017;2017. doi:10.1155/2017/8416763

16. Ahmad A, Singhal U, Hossain MM, Islam N, Rizvi I. The role of the endogenous antioxidant enzymes and malondialdehyde in essential hypertension. *Journal of Clinical and Diagnostic Research*. 2013;7(6):987-990. doi:10.7860/JCDR/2013/5829.3091

17. Gu JW, Liu JH, Xiao HN, et al. Relationship between plasma levels of 25-hydroxyvitamin D and arterial stiffness in elderly Chinese with non-dipper hypertension: An observational study. *Medicine (United States)*. 2020;99(7):e19200-e19200.

doi:10.1097/MD.0000000000019200

18. Cheng J, Wang F, Yu DF, Wu PF, Chen JG. The cytotoxic mechanism of malondialdehyde and protective effect of carnosine via protein cross-linking/mitochondrial dysfunction/reactive oxygen species/MAPK pathway in neurons. *European Journal of Pharmacology*. 2011;650(1):184-194. doi:10.1016/j.ejphar.2010.09.033

19. Wu G. *Important Roles of Dietary Taurine, Creatine, Carnosine, Anserine and 4-Hydroxyproline in Human Nutrition and Health*. Vol 52. Springer Vienna; 2020. doi:10.1007/s00726-020-02823-6

20. Meng X, Li Y, Li S, et al. Dietary sources and bioactivities of melatonin. *Nutrients*. 2017;9(4):367. doi:10.3390/nu9040367

21. Tordjman S, Chokron S, Delorme R, et al. Melatonin: Pharmacology, Functions and Therapeutic Benefits. *Current Neuropharmacology*. 2017;15(3):434-443. doi:10.2174/1570159x14666161228122115

22. Mokhtari V, Afsharian P, Shahhoseini M, Kalantar SM, Moini A. A review on various uses of N-acetyl cysteine. *Cell Journal*. 2017;19(1):11-17. doi:10.22074/cellj.2016.4872

23. Cai JG, Luo LM, Tang H, Zhou L. Cytotoxicity of Malondialdehyde and Cytoprotective Effects of Taurine via Oxidative Stress and PGC-1α Signal Pathway in C2C12 Cells. *Molecular Biology*. 2018;52(4):532-542. doi:10.1134/S0026898418040043

24. Peluso M, Munnia A, Piro S, et al. Fruit and vegetable and fried food consumption and 3-(2-deoxy-β-D- erythro-pentafuranosyl)pyrimido[1,2-α] purin-10(3H)-one deoxyguanosine adduct formation. *Free Radical Research*. 2012;46(1):85-92. doi:10.3109/10715762.2011.640676

25. Saieva C, Peluso M, Palli D, et al. Dietary and lifestyle determinants of malondialdehyde DNA adducts in a representative sample of the Florence City population. *Mutagenesis*. 2016;31(4):475-480. doi:10.1093/mutage/gew012

Chapter 11: Protocol

What gets measured gets managed.

Although everything in this book is just a hypothesis, maybe confirmed in different multiple papers. There is a need for clinical measurement. High-performance liquid chromatography with/without fluorescence detection is economically feasible, rapid, and can be clinically conducted.

Redox markers:

1. Malondialdehyde levels: Depends on genetic as well as behavioral factors. Here, this behavioral factor can be decreased as much as possible and may decrease the predisposition of genetic factors to behavioral stress.
2. 3-nitro tyrosine: Genetically-equipped individuals tolerate higher levels. Refer external interventions for lowering 3NT plasma values.
3. Lycopene: refer dietary intervention
4. Alpha-tocopherol: refer dietary intervention
5. Cysteine: refer dietary intervention

Reference methods:

1. Make use of standard deviations (this method will take time to be implemented).
2. Mean method:
    a. Take reference values during adolescence (13-18 years), the age group of highest

physical attributes, and try to reach these values. It would be better if desired interventions are given for a minimum duration to elicit a significant desired response, i.e.15-30 days.
b. In absence of age reference values, take plasma values of
   i. Adolescent son and daughter, and then take their mean. slightly adjusting for male or female values.
   ii. Pedigree chart based closest adolescent age group values that can be available.
   (NOTE: MDA also takes into account lifestyle like smoking, drinking, eating habits; this mean method can help evaluate for behavioral oxidative stress, by referencing with close working colleagues as well. However, the clinical significance in such a scenario is dubious but an individual pathological correction may need it.)

Now, a comparison of present values and reference values will decide the priority of interventions among the five redox markers. Then, interventions approach the reference values and follow up of plasma levels on regular testing. Unlike other clinical tests, here values are seen in relative terms and not to be stubborn to obtain values within a fixed range. This relative change in plasma level, increase or decrease as desirable for different redox markers provides information on strength of safety net. The higher the change in values seen, the stronger will be the safety net against mortality or severe morbidity.

Chapter 12: FUTURE PROSPECTS

A clinical trial to formulate the ideal dosage, and also confirm the extent to which it will be beneficial is needed. Although, combining this approach with the existing medical practice against COVID19 infection will provide better treatment, but to what extent will need to be established.

Few steps in the above-mentioned approach, despite being a good adaptation, higher 3-nitro tyrosine is indicating higher oxidative stress. Only because, tyrosine radical formation is a good step for biological functions, the cost is oxidative damage. A detailed account will be needed to evaluate, and formulate a precise method of attenuation. Oxidative stress-induced damage is an ongoing process, and simply managing it is a slower method. It can be further accelerated, as we should consider cellular clearing mechanisms of residuals like Advanced Glycation End Products, Advanced Lipoxidation End Products, and other outcomes of reactive species like, Reactive Carbonyl Species, Reactive Oxygen Species, Reactive Nitrogen Species, etc., instead of simply decreasing their production.

Chapter 13: Need for universal therapy

With the advancement of medical knowledge, improving the health status of every individual has increased the global life expectancy and quality of life. However, after a significant time interval, we are always presented with different types of pathologies, which have no existing cure. For instance, AIDS used to mean end-of-life disorder, now we have medication that may not render you a negative report, but will allow you to sustain a healthy life. We also have diseases like pancreatic carcinoma, the disease itself is diagnosed way too late, and mostly accidentally, such that saving a life is not possible because of delayed diagnosis. There are severe complications of different diseases, acute emergencies, which are usually characterized by increased redox stress.

Maybe nullifying this redox stress will delay the pathological outcome, buy more time for the treatments to work, and ultimately avoid mortality. And a similar analogy for chronic diseases, as aging is a major risk factor; avoiding the accumulation of toxic metabolic wastes, again safety against chronic diseases. And for diseases where aging is not a major risk factor, health, not the immune status is questionable. And as discussed earlier, if we can improve health as a whole, instead of the immune system alone, some benefits may be presented.

Average life expectancy is increasing worldwide, however, Japan's life expectancy is higher than the rest of the world. It is consequence of their dietary, behavioral, and environmental factors. Now, living in an environment that makes you work harder, also increases life expectancy, but not hitting the gym. If it is possible to slow down the accumulated impairment over time, life span is elongated; and when nullified, death may be a choice.

This theory is probably still incomplete, lacking the precise quantification of modern medicine, but is highly feasible, and thus, modern medicine needs to confirm or deny via clinical trials but ultimately create a universal treatment for all diseases.

An incentive to complete this task-

"No doctor has ever told me that antioxidants itself can have a significant change of health status. But, we use lycopene for prostate hypertrophy an age-related disorder, cysteine was part of the treatment regimen in only known cured case of AIDS, melatonin is used as adjunctive therapy in thyroid carcinoma, there are research papers requesting carnosine and taurine be made part of essential nutrients, resveratrol acts on sirtuin receptors which is an established anti-aging receptor! Everything sounds too good to be true, so combine them all, maybe we can have a better answer. Well, it's all just a theory, neither the author is credible enough nor the description is detailed enough. But then again, the history of medical science is not exactly a tale of goodness. We have approved treatments for far less."

www.ingramcontent.com/pod-product-compliance
Lightning Source LLC
Chambersburg PA
CBHW070826220526
45466CB00002B/763